ConstipatedKIDS.com

BedwettingAndAccidents.com

Jane and the Giant Poop, 1st Edition
Text Copyright © 2017 Steve J. Hodges and Suzanne Schlosberg
Illustration Copyright © 2017 Cristina Acosta
Book design: DyanRothDesign.com

O'regan press

Library of Congress Cataloging-in-Publication Data is available on file.

ISBN: 978-0-9908774-4-8

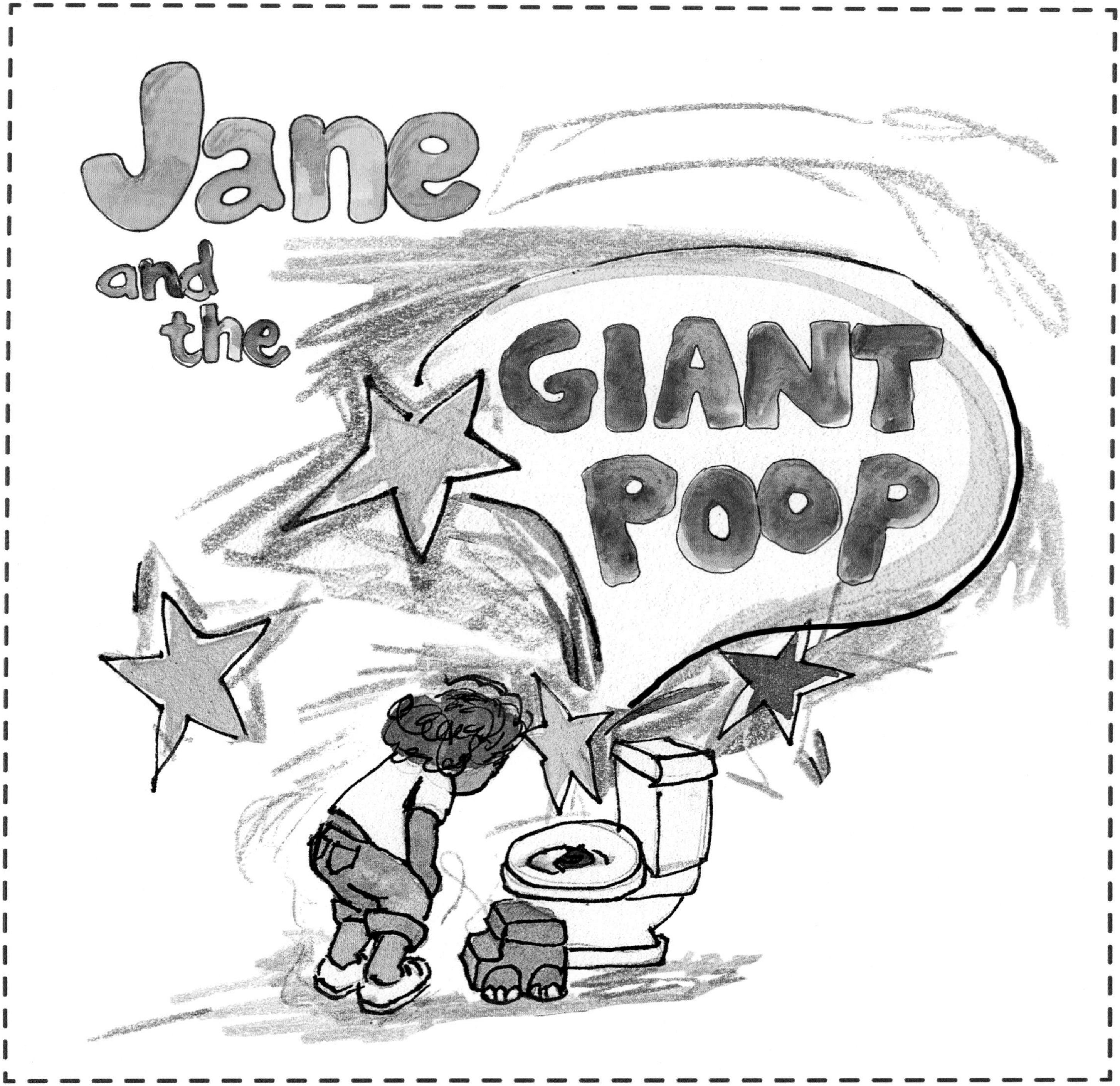
Jane
and the
GIANT
POOP

Cast of Characters

Jane

Jane is a strong girl who loves to do karate, ride her scooter, and tell jokes. But lately she hasn't been feeling like her happy self. It hurts for her to poop, and often she has to pee really badly. Sometimes her poops are huge; other times they are small and hard, like marbles or rabbit pellets. Jane and her mom are on a mission to solve her problem!

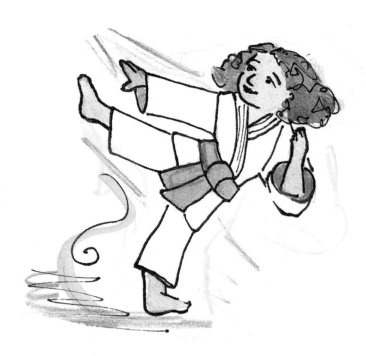

Dr. Pooper

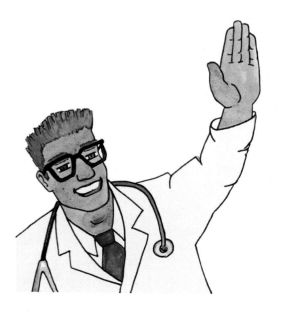

Dr. Pooper is a real doctor! That isn't his real name, but it's what his patients call him because his job is to help kids who have trouble with pooping and peeing.

Millions of children all over the world have toileting difficulties. For some kids, pooping hurts. Others get stomachaches. Still other kids wet the bed or have pee or poop accidents during the day.

If you have toilet troubles, like Jane, Dr. Pooper wants you to know: It's not your fault! Children never have potty problems on purpose. It just means your insides have gone a little nutty. But don't worry: The problems can be fixed!

The Colon and Rectum

Your **colon** is a tube in your belly where poop gets made; it's like a poop factory. Your **rectum** is the end of your colon; it's where poop hangs out before you let it out of your bottom.

Here's how your poop factory works: After you chew your food, the mashed-up bits travel down a tube and into your stomach, where it gets mashed into smaller bits. Then, these tiny bits move into a long, twisty tube called the small intestine. Some of the mashed-up food passes through the walls of this tube into your body, to give you energy and keep you healthy. The bits your body doesn't need travel on to your colon to become poop!

If you don't let poop out every day, it starts piling up and hardening in your rectum. When the poop pile gets super big, it stretches your rectum, the way a snake's belly stretches after the snake eats a rat for dinner! But snake bellies are supposed to stretch; rectums aren't.

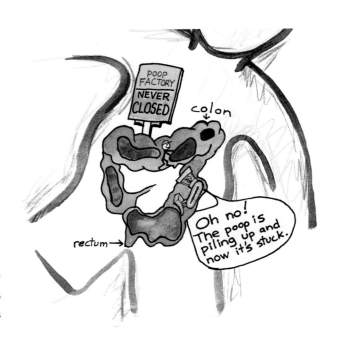

The Bladder

Your bladder is a stretchy bag that holds your pee. Depending on your age, your bladder could be the size of an orange or the size of a cantaloupe. When you drink a beverage or eat watery foods, your bladder starts to fill up. When it gets full enough, it sends a signal to your brain that tells you: *It's time to pee!*

Your bladder sits really close to your rectum, the tube that holds poop before you let it out. So when your rectum gets overstuffed with poop, it starts squishing your bladder. This makes your bladder wacky! You might feel like you need to pee RIGHT THIS MINUTE! You might even have a pee accident.

To keep your bladder healthy, it's important to poop every day and pee every few hours.

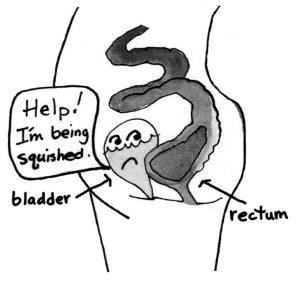

3

Once there was a potty
that got terribly clogged
by an extra-large poop
that resembled a log.

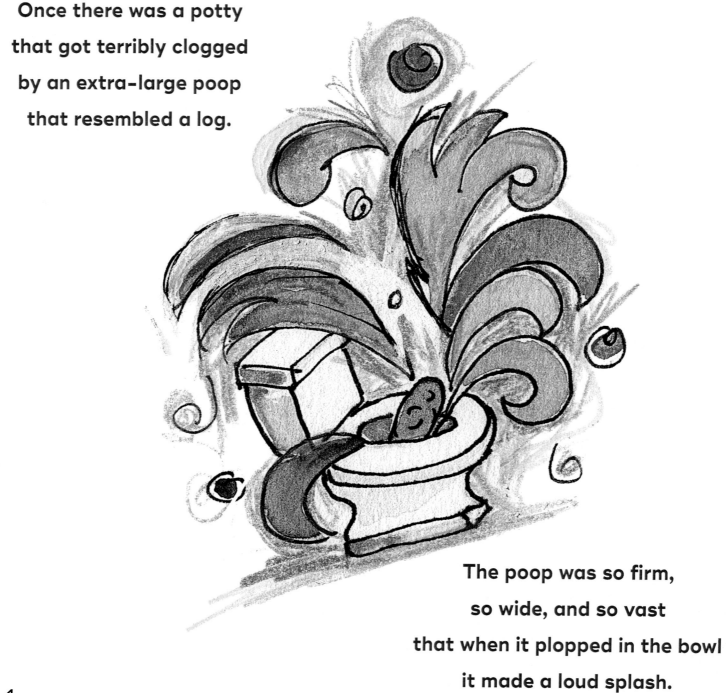

The poop was so firm,
so wide, and so vast
that when it plopped in the bowl
it made a loud splash.

The pooper was Jane,
a strong girl who said,
"Pooping is hard!"
and almost turned red.

When Jane was done wiping
she pressed down the lever,
but the toilet wouldn't flush —
it was a useless endeavor.

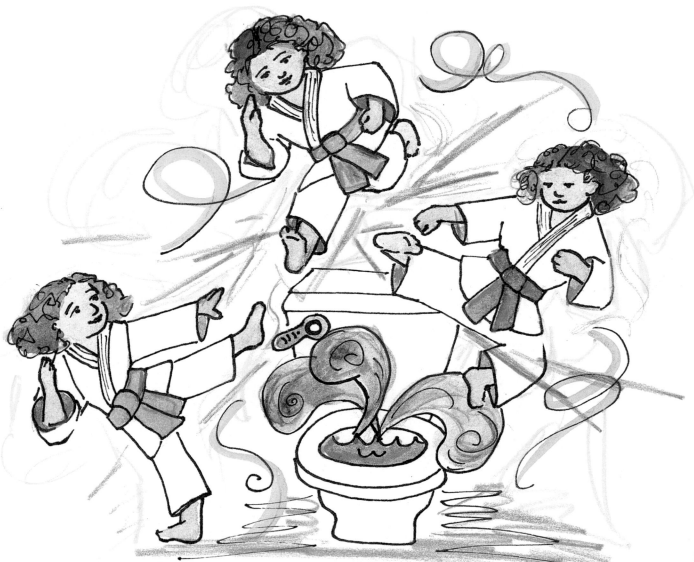

5

Jane called for her mom
to come fix the blockage.
"Holy cow!" her mom cried.
"It's a jumbo sausage!"

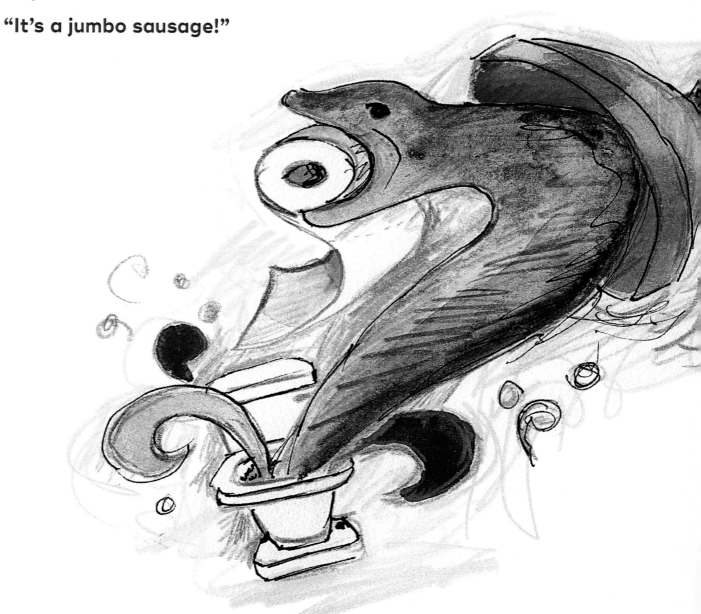

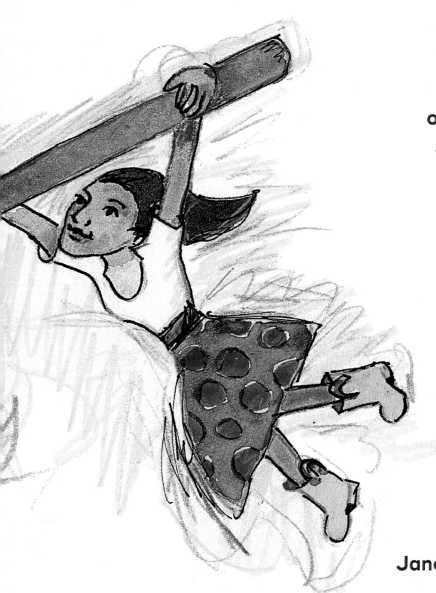

Jane's dad was in awe
of what Jane could produce.
"That's larger than mine —
snake on the loose!"

Jane inspected the log
and started to wonder
if the family should call
Paulie the plumber.

"No, I'll get the plunger,"
Jane's mom assured her daughter.
"It won't be a problem
to restore the water."

It was not the first time
Jane's poop had been plump.
For months on end, logs had
been exiting her rump.

"My stomach hurts!"
Jane would complain.
And each time she pooped,
she said she felt pain.

A genial jokester,
Jane was normally sunny.
"Your fly's down!"
she'd say, just to be funny.

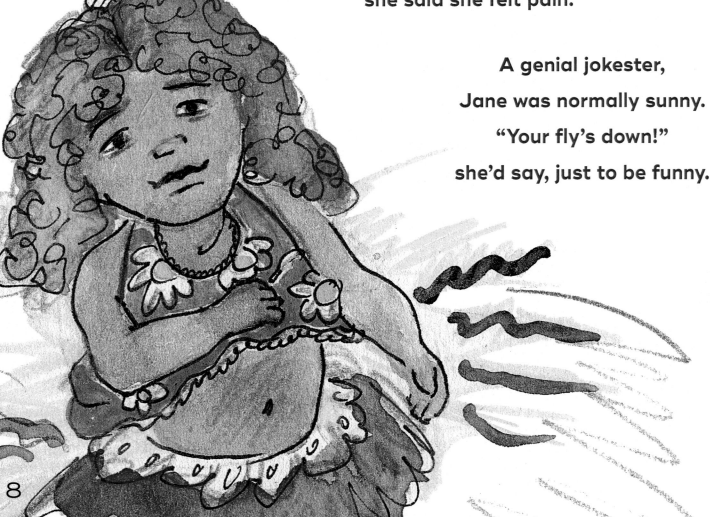

8

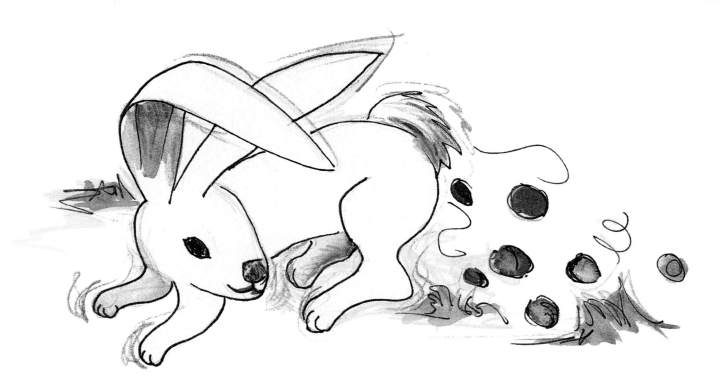

But Jane hadn't been herself since pooping got tough.
She didn't feel like joking and sometimes was gruff.

On quite a few days
Jane did not poop at all,
and on other days,
her poops came out small.

Some looked like marbles — dark, round, and hard —
or pellets from the bunny that lived in Jane's yard.

9

Jane drove with her mom
to see Dr. Pooper,
who explained that hard poops
are not at all super.

"Lots of folks think
a big log is just fine.
However, it's actually
a great big sign."

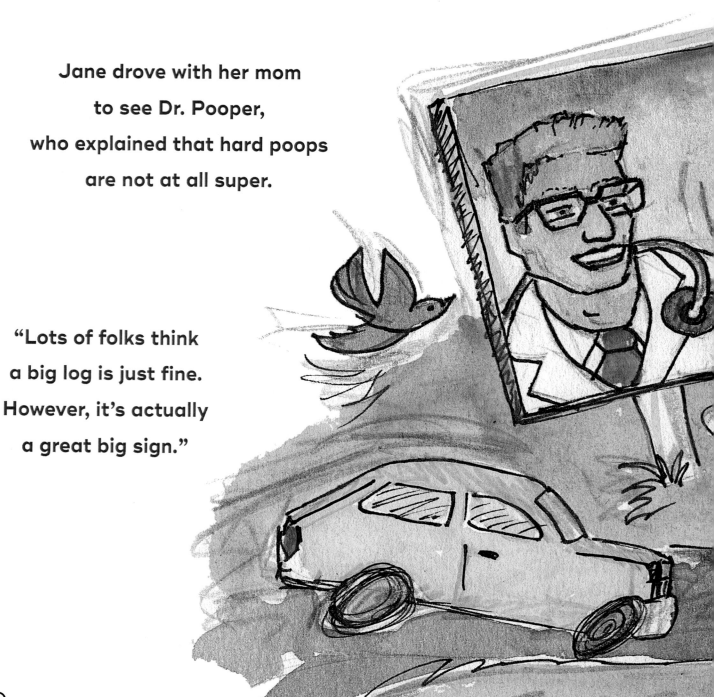

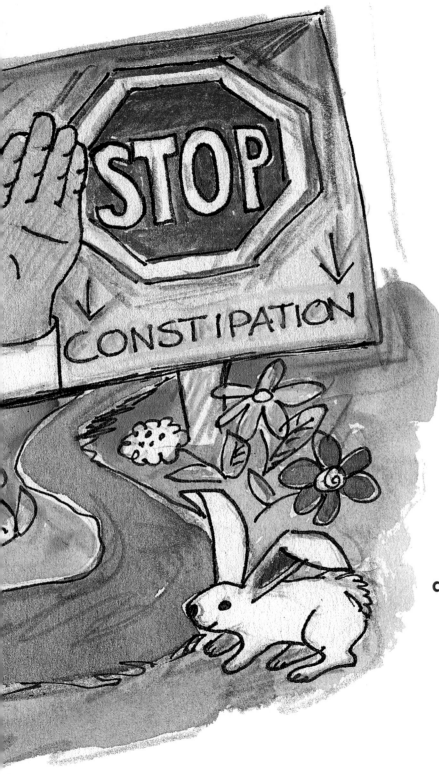

"It means poop has piled
up at the end of your colon,
in a place called the rectum,
which becomes stretched
and swollen."

"A pile-up of poop
is called 'constipation,'
and happens to kids every day,
not just on vacation."

11

When a clogged-up rectum
becomes wider and fatter,
it can, the doc said,
press on your bladder.

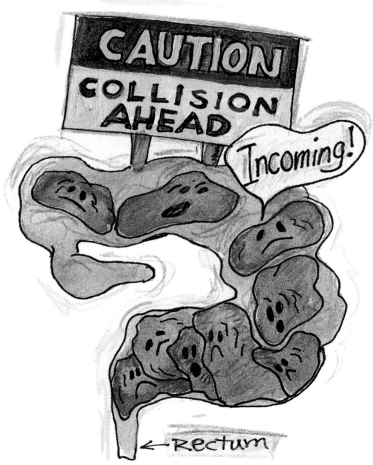

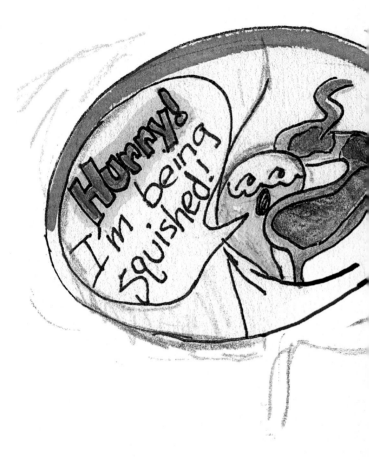

"A squished bladder can hiccup
and leak overnight
or during the day
when you're flying a kite."

"A bladder that's squished
can get grouchy and mad,
which makes children say,
'I have to pee REALLY bad!'"

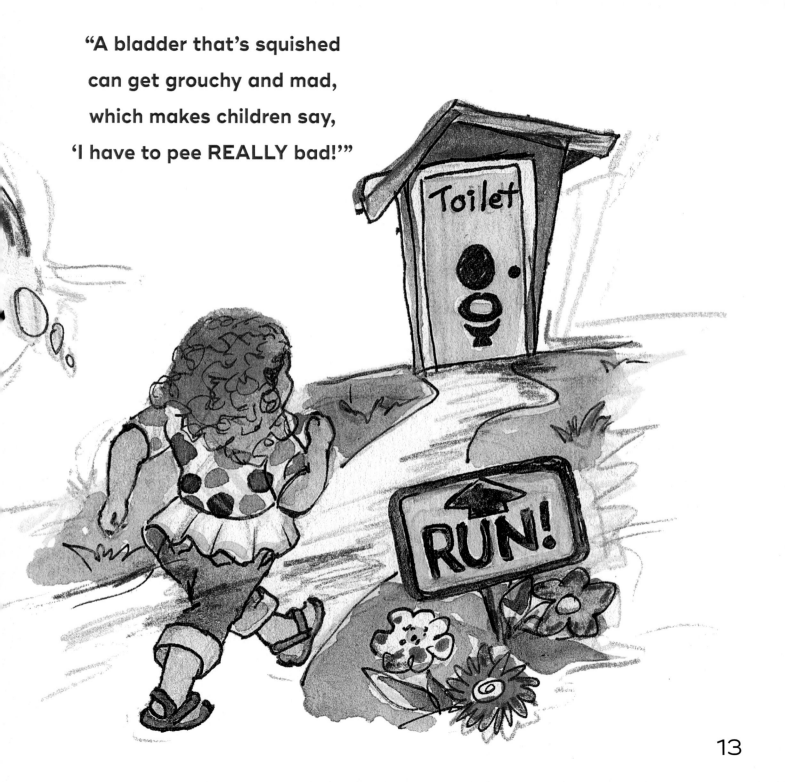

But most common of all
is what Jane had been feeling:
an ache in her belly
that was not receding.

"I knew," said Jane's mom,
"her poop had been sporadic,
but I had no clue constipation
could wreak so much havoc."

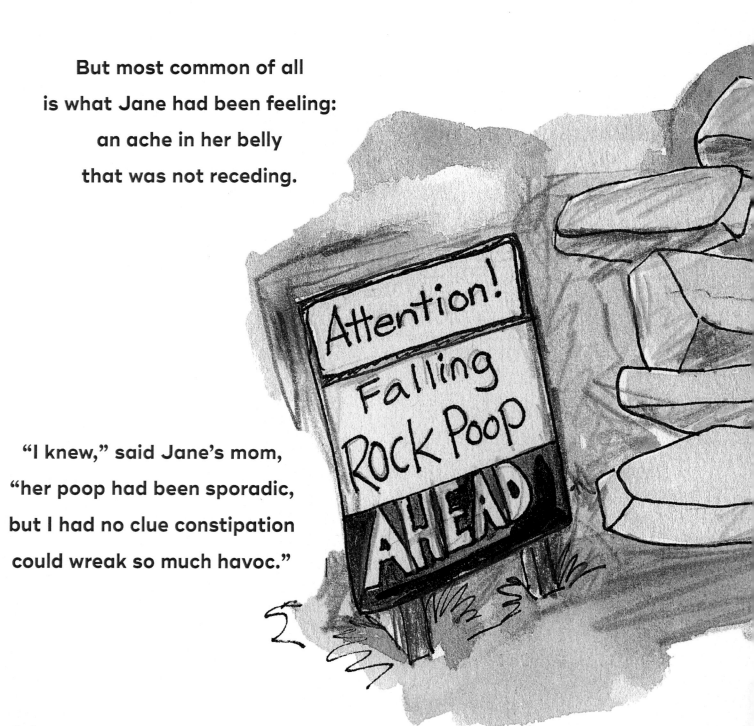

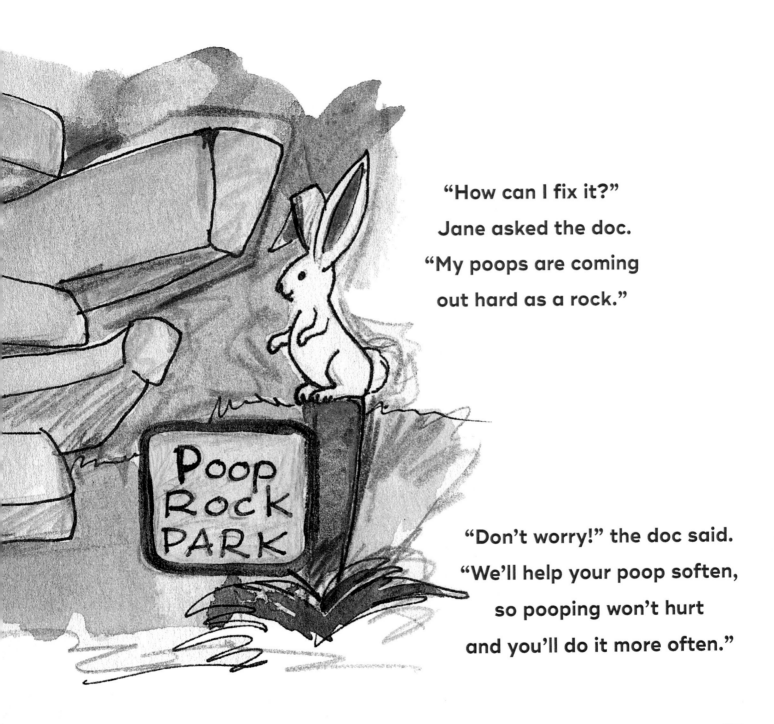

"How can I fix it?"
Jane asked the doc.
"My poops are coming
out hard as a rock."

"Don't worry!" the doc said.
"We'll help your poop soften,
so pooping won't hurt
and you'll do it more often."

Dr. Pooper handed Jane
his favorite chart,
which shows six kinds of poop,
a work of fine art!

"Healthy poop is a blob,
not formed in a shape.
It's like pudding," the doc said,
"not a log or a grape."

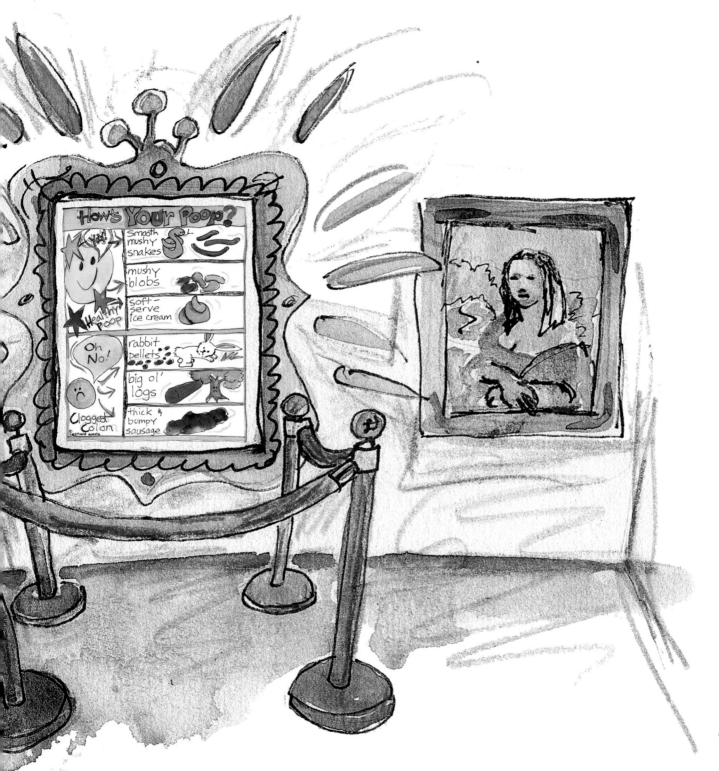

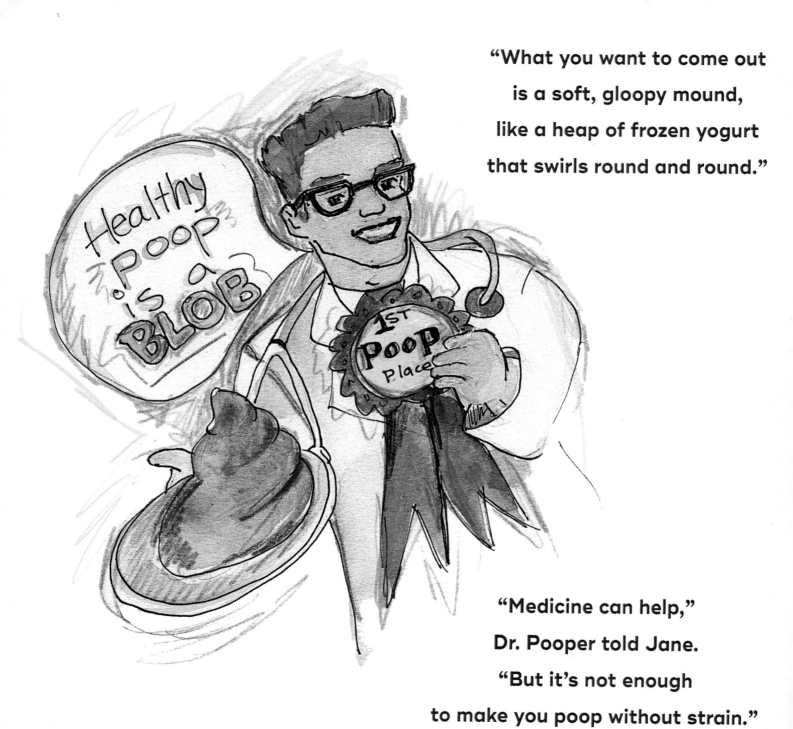

"What you want to come out
is a soft, gloopy mound,
like a heap of frozen yogurt
that swirls round and round."

"Medicine can help,"
Dr. Pooper told Jane.
"But it's not enough
to make you poop without strain."

18

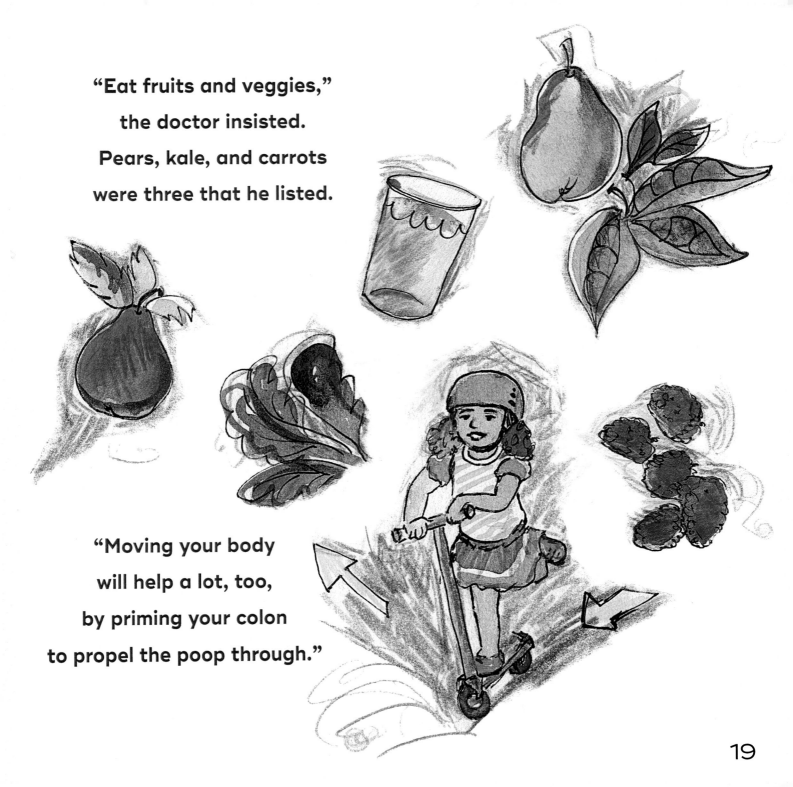

"Eat fruits and veggies,"
the doctor insisted.
Pears, kale, and carrots
were three that he listed.

"Moving your body
will help a lot, too,
by priming your colon
to propel the poop through."

19

"Ride a bike, if you like, or go for a jog.
Play ball, climb a wall, or walk with your dog."

"I like to jump rope," Jane told her physician,
"and I can do yoga — most any position!"

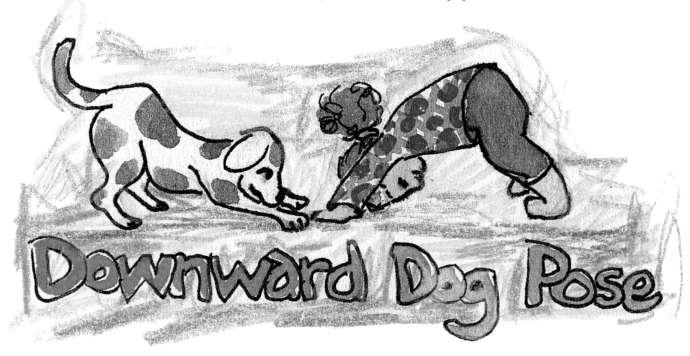

Downward Dog Pose

Dr. Pooper advised Jane to poop every day,
so her colon would empty without a delay.

"But what if," Jane asked, "I don't need to go?"
"If you don't try," said the doc, "you won't truly know."

"The best time to poop
is right after you eat.
And it's best if you sit
with a stool under your feet."

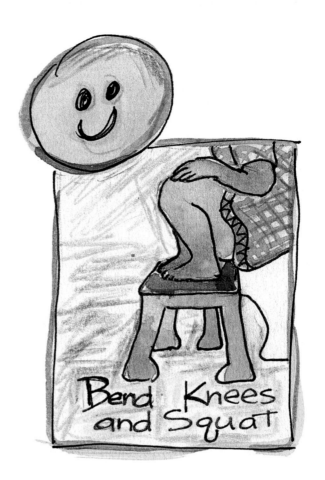

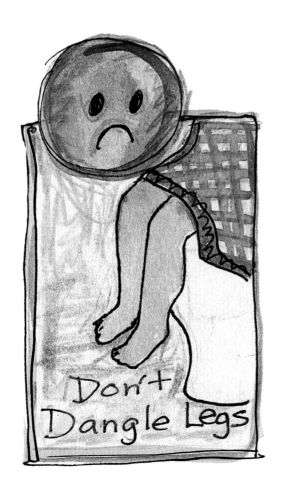

"If your legs hang," the doc said,
"your potty muscles tense.
So you can't fully relax
and make pooping commence."

"But when you try pooping
with your legs in a squat,
poop slides right out
and plops in the pot."

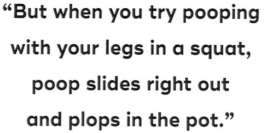

"Leaning forward helps, too,
elbows on knees.
Keep those legs wide apart
to make pooping a breeze!"

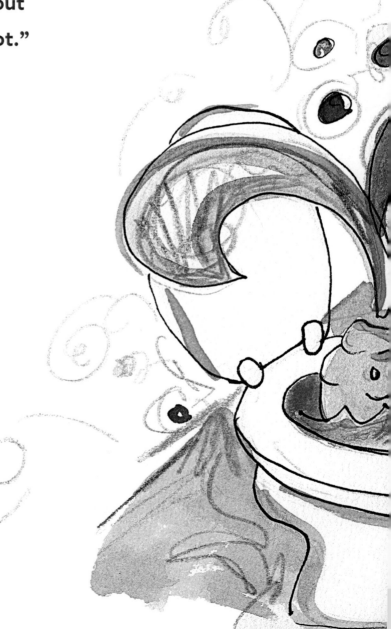

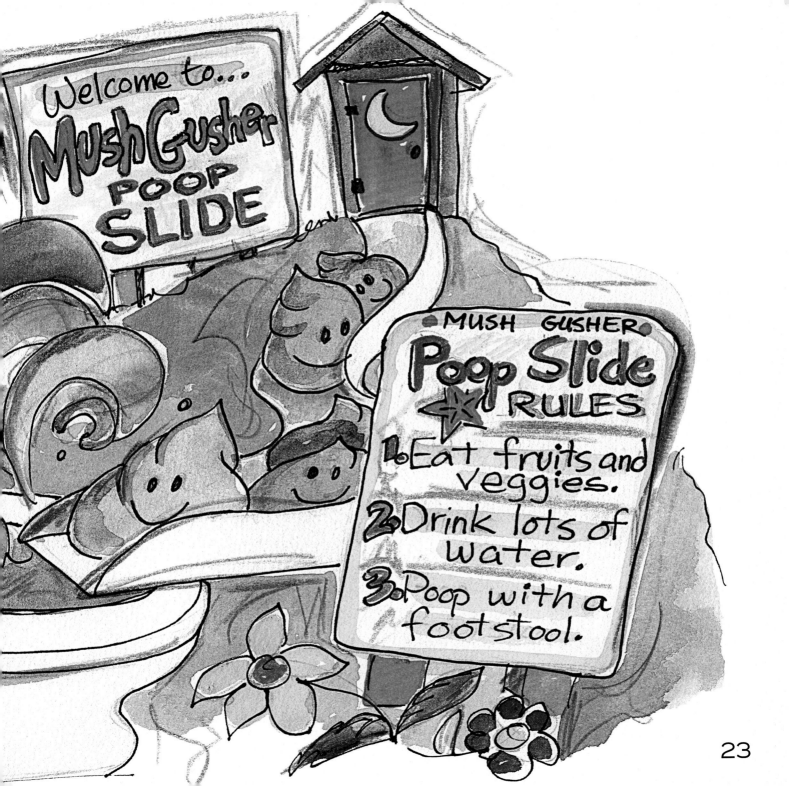

23

Jane swam and did yoga,
and jumped lots of rope.
She ate beans and zucchini
and ripe cantaloupe.

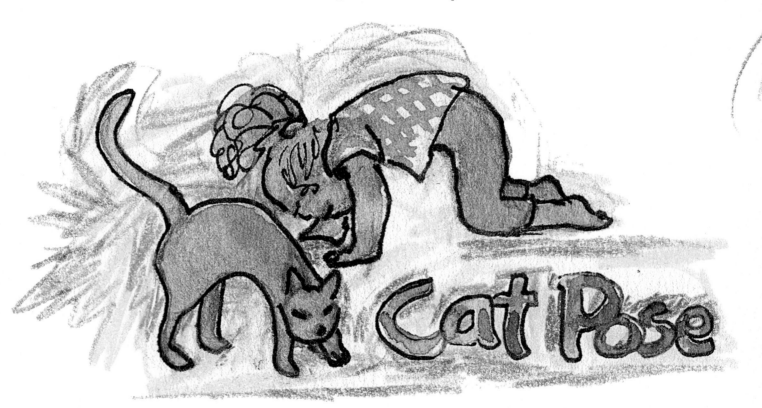

She made a habit of using
the bathroom at school,
once her mom asked the teacher
to make flexible rules.

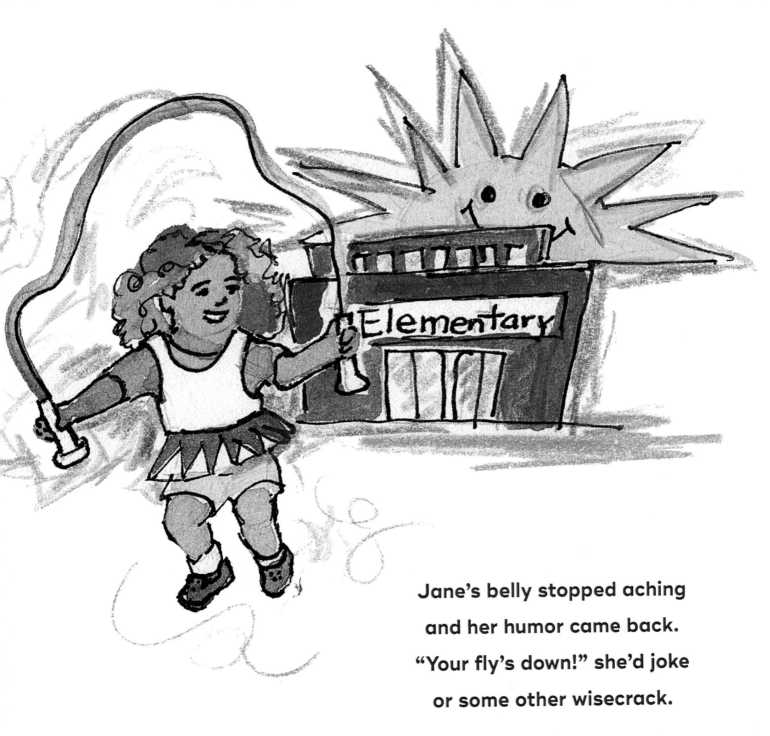

Jane's belly stopped aching
and her humor came back.
"Your fly's down!" she'd joke
or some other wisecrack.

Whenever Jane pooped,
she peered into the bowl.
And she'd announce to her mom
when she'd reached her goal.

"Hooray!" she'd shout
after inspecting her pile.
"It looks like a milkshake —
my best in a while!"

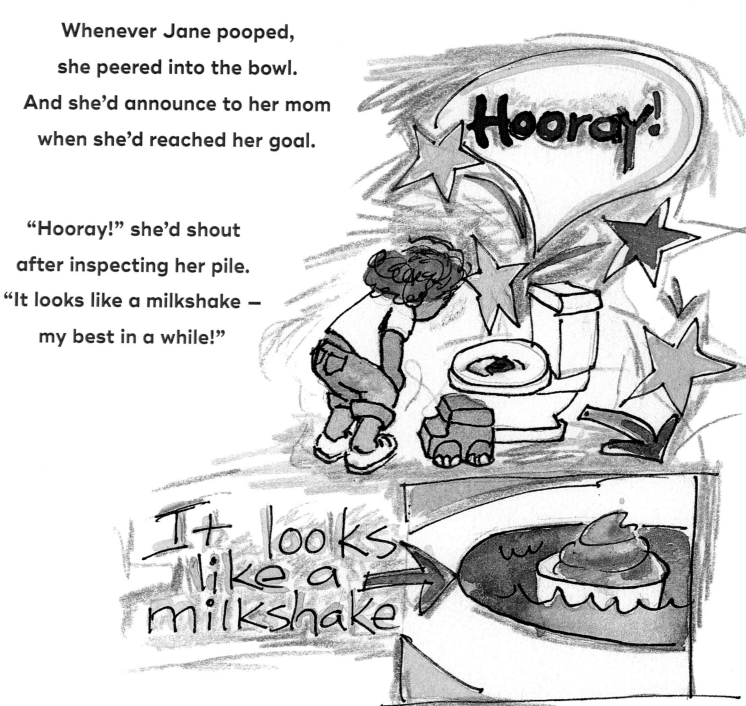

Jane was proud when she'd poop
a squishy cow patty.
"I bet it's softer than yours!"
she'd say to her daddy.

It wasn't long before
Jane's poop turned to mush.
And forever after,
the toilet would flush.

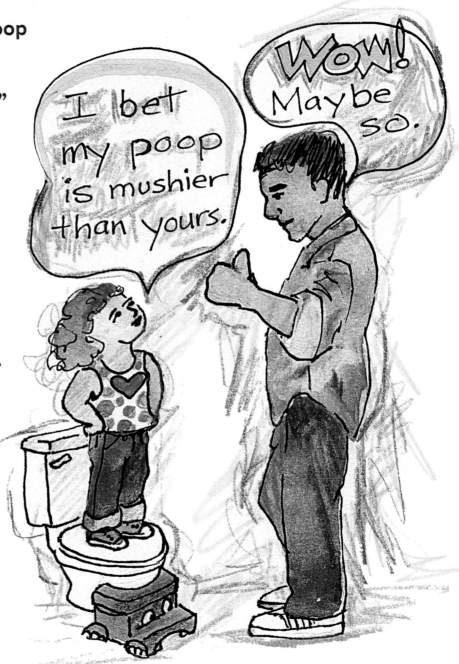

27

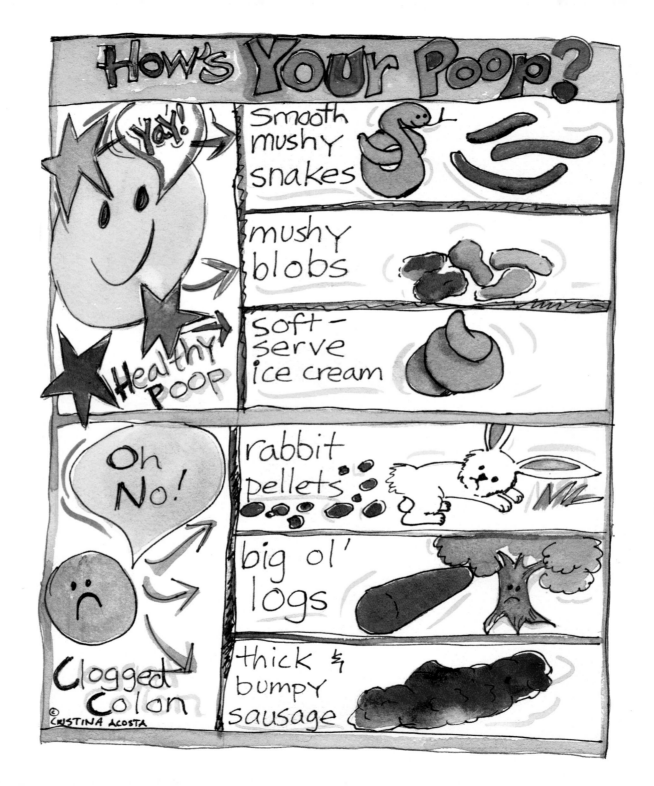

12 Signs

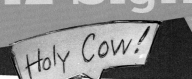

Your Child is Constipated

1 **XXL poops.** We're talking "Holy cow!" poops — larger than ¾" x 6."

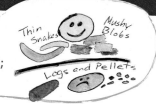

2 **Firm poops.** Logs or pellets = bad; thin snakes or mushy blobs = good.

3 **Poop accidents.** When the rectum is overstuffed, poop just falls out.

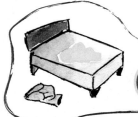

4 **Bedwetting and pee accidents.** A big ol' poop mass squishes the bladder.

5 **Recurrent UTIs.** Bacteria from overflowing poop crawl up to the bladder.

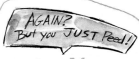

6 **Extremely frequent and/or urgent peeing.** You think, "AGAIN? But you JUST peed!"

7 **Infrequent pooping.** But daily pooping doesn't rule out constipation.

8 **Pooping more than 2x/day.** A stretched-out rectum lacks the tone to evacuate fully.

9 **Belly pain.** Constipation is the #1 source of tummy ache in kids.

10 **Skid marks or itchy anus.** Clogged kids can't fully empty → bottom is hard to wipe → poop stains.

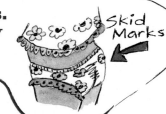

11 **Super-loose poop.** Some poop can ooze around the large, hard rectal clog.

12 **Continued trouble toilet training.** Your child may fear pooping or hide to poop in diapers.

The Story Behind
Jane and the Giant Poop

Q&A with Steve Hodges, M.D.

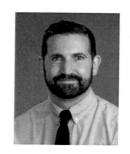

Associate Professor of Pediatric Urology, Wake Forest University School of Medicine

Co-author, *The M.O.P. Book*, *It's No Accident*, and *Bedwetting and Accidents Aren't Your Fault*

Q: What inspired you to write *Jane and the Giant Poop*?

A: I'm a goofball at heart, and I was looking for a fun and slightly outrageous way to bring attention to our childhood constipation epidemic. Children in the developed world have exceedingly high rates of constipation, up to 30% in some populations, studies show, though I suspect that's an underestimation. Constipation is a misunderstood condition with a high recurrence rate. Problems often follow these kids into adulthood.

The signs of constipation in children (see page 31) can be subtle and are unknown to many families and physicians. So even severely constipated children often go undiagnosed and untreated.

Though constipation is typically defined as "pooping less than 3 times a week," this is a highly misleading definition. Many severely constipated children poop daily, even two or three times a day, because they never fully empty. Sure, they're "regular," but their rectums are also clogged. It's important for parents and medical providers to look beyond frequency when assessing whether a child is constipated. Kids can learn the signs, too!

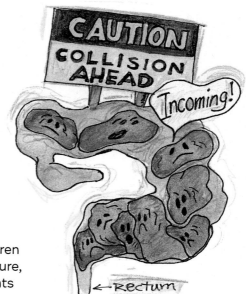

The signs of a poop pile-up are often subtle.

Q: You're a pediatric urologist — why are you writing about constipation?

A: Because constipation is the cause of virtually all the urological problems I treat: bedwetting, daytime accidents, recurrent urinary tract infections, and urinary urgency and frequency. Constipation triggers urinary troubles because the bladder sits right near the rectum. When poop piles up, it forms a large, hard mass that stretches the rectum (think: rat in a snake's belly) and presses against and aggravates the bladder.

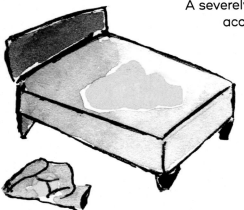

A severely clogged rectum is also the only cause, in healthy children, of poop accidents (encopresis). In children with encopresis, the stretched rectum has lost tone and sensation, so poop doesn't move along well and may fall out of the child's bottom without the child even noticing. These kids don't sense the need to poop, so even more stool piles up, perpetuating a vicious cycle. Most of my encopresis patients also have urinary problems.

The connection between constipation and wetting (enuresis) is well documented in the scientific literature (see the Research page at BedwettingAndAccidents.com), and it's confirmed daily in my practice. X-rays of my wetting patients show that nearly all of them are severely constipated. Often I see a softball-sized stool mass flattening the bladder.

Constipation causes bedwetting because the rectum sits so close to the bladder.

Many parents are stunned by the films — they had no idea their child was even constipated. X-rays help families realize that bedwetting is in no way the child's fault and has nothing to do with "deep sleep," "hormonal imbalances," or an "underdeveloped" bladder.

When children get cleaned out on a daily basis, their stretched rectums shrink back to size and stop bothering the bladder, and accidents resolve. I hope *Jane and the Giant Poop* will prompt families to detect and treat constipation before serious toileting difficulties develop.

Q: Why are so many children constipated?

A: My research and clinical practice point to three main reasons:

1.) The highly processed Western diet: The same eating habits driving the childhood obesity epidemic cause firm stools and painful pooping. Many babies become constipated upon starting solids, and poop piles up from there. In some children, intolerances or allergies to foods such as dairy or wheat can trigger constipation.

2.) Early toilet training: Because of preschool requirements, many parents potty train their children as toddlers. Problem is, 2-year-olds generally don't have the judgment to respond to their bodies' urges in a timely manner, so many of them develop the holding habit. My most severely constipated patients tend to be those who potty trained earliest; in other words, they've been in charge of their toileting the longest.

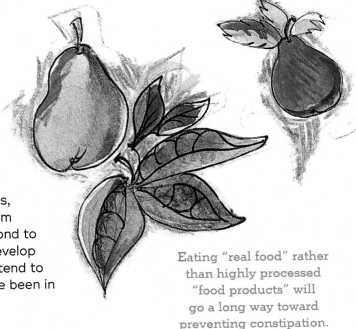

Eating "real food" rather than highly processed "food products" will go a long way toward preventing constipation.

31

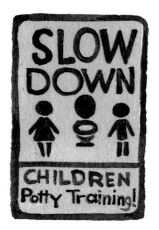

Let go of deadlines and expectations for potty training

In a study published in *Research and Reports in Urology*, my clinic found that children trained before age 2 have triple the risk of developing constipation and wetting problems compared with children trained later. I advise training around age 3, though maturity is more important than age. Still, even when children are ready to use the toilet, potty training is prime time for constipation to develop. Parents and teachers must vigilantly watch for the signs. When children have trouble graduating to "fully" trained, it's because they are too young to train, are constipated, or both.

3.) Restrictive school bathroom policies: Countless schools promote constipation and bladder problems by rewarding students who don't use bathroom passes or punishing those who do. A University of California at San Francisco survey, published in the *Journal of Urology*, found that 76% of elementary school teachers set bathroom policies that may compromise their students' urinary health.

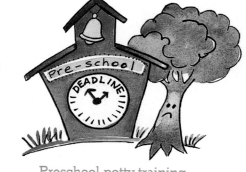

Preschool potty-training requirements prompt many parents to train their children before they are truly ready.

Compounding the problem, many K-12 students never use school bathrooms because they are grossed out by unclean conditions or afraid of being bullied. I have many patients who literally never pee or poop at school; they may go from 7:30 a.m. to 3:30 p.m. without using the toilet. Holding pee exacerbates the problems caused by holding poop.

Ask your children how often they use the toilet at school, and find out what may be stopping them, whether it's a classroom policy, fear, or embarrassment. Most teachers will make accommodations if you ask. You can educate teachers and administrators with "The K-12 Teacher's Fact Sheet on Childhood Toileting Troubles," available free at BedwettingAndAccidents.com.

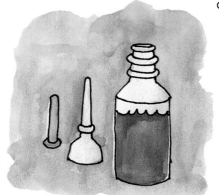

Enemas are the most effective way to treat chronic constipation in children who have accidents.

Q: What's the best way to treat constipation?

A: Aggressively! Constipation in children is often perceived as a minor nuisance and is typically undertreated by doctors. By the time adults recognize a child is constipated, the child's pipes may have been clogged for months, if not years. At this point the child needs vigorous measures — such as laxatives, suppositories, and/or enemas — to clean out the stuffed, stretched rectum

It is certainly important for children to eat "real" food instead of highly processed "food products," stay active, and drink plenty of water. However, lifestyle measures often are not sufficient to resolve constipation, especially in children who have difficulty potty training and in toiled-trained children who have accidents or wet the bed. All the prunes in the world won't dislodge a softball-sized mass of stool stretching the rectum.

For children who have accidents, enemas are the most effective treatment. (And yes, they're safe.) While some adults consider it "unnatural" to give a child enemas, suppositories, or laxatives, I would argue that it is unnatural — and harmful in numerous ways — for a child to carry around a belly full of poop.

Holding poop is a deeply ingrained habit. Once pooping becomes painful for children, they tend to maintain that "pooping equals pain" association, even long after pooping ceases to be uncomfortable. To break this association and prevent a recurrence, children need extended treatment. Once your child no longer shows signs of constipation — that means she's pooping big piles of mush every day — you may need to stick with treatment for months or longer.

I offer specific treatment recommendations, based on a child's age and symptoms, at BedwettingAndAccidents.com and ConstipatedKids.com.

Many doctors may rely too heavily on Miralax to resolve constipation.

Q: Miralax is the most popular constipation medication for kids. Do you think it could be toxic?

A: I think Miralax and its generic equivalents (powders containing PEG 3350) are safe for children, but there are alternatives, such as lactulose and magnesium citrate, that do the same job and pose no safety concerns at all. Parents worried about Miralax should know they have other options.

The U.S. Food and Drug Administration has commissioned researchers to study whether PEG 3350 may trigger psychiatric symptoms, such as aggression, phobias, and mood swings. I eagerly await the results of this study, but I suspect the researchers won't find a connection. Search for my blog post "Is Miralax Poisoning Children?" for an in-depth discussion of Miralax safety.

At this point my concern about PEG 3350 is not that the drug is poisonous; it's that physicians over-rely on it to treat chronic constipation. Countless children who take Miralax really need suppositories and/or enemas. Simply softening a child's stool, which is what Miralax accomplishes, isn't enough for many children. Often, stool softened by PEG 3350 just oozes around the hardened mass. The child appears to be pooping more, but nothing inside has changed. In some kids, Miralax can make matters worse, triggering poop accidents that weren't happening before.

Prior to landing in my clinic, most of my enuresis and encopresis patients were prescribed nothing but Miralax. And when Miralax failed to resolve the problem, these kids were prescribed . . . more Miralax. And then more!

Learn more about constipation at BedwettingAndAccidents.com and ConstipatedKIDS.com.

Praise for Our Other Books!

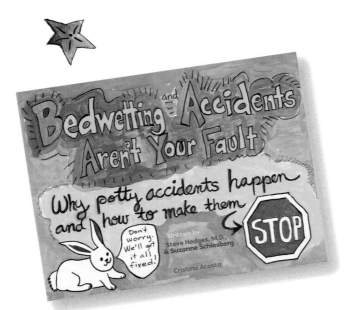

Praise for
Bedwetting and Accidents Aren't Your Fault

"**Every family dealing with accidents or bedwetting should own this engaging and eye-opening book!**"
– *Amy McCready, founder of Positive Parenting Solutions and author of If I Have to Tell You One More Time...*

"**Finally – an entertaining, encouraging book about potty problems! I've dreamed about showing illustrations like these to my patients.**"
– *Angelique Champeau, NP, Director, Pediatric Continence Clinic, UCSF Benioff Children's Hospital, Oakland and San Francisco*

"**Terrific! The illustrations are so much fun they remove any possible embarrassment, and the tone is friendly and supportive.**"
– *Laura Markham, Ph.D., author of Peaceful Parent, Happy Kids: How to Stop Yelling and Start Connecting*

Dr. Pooper is a ROCKSTAR!!! I'd remind my son, "What does Dr. Pooper want you to do every day?" and that would convince him to give it a try!
—*Amazon verified purchaser*

Praise for
The M.O.P. Book

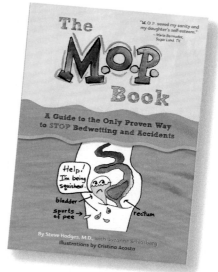

"**M.O.P. works radically better than anything else.**"

– *James Sander, MD, Director of Pediatric Urology*
Doctors Hospital at Renaissance, Edinburg, TX

"**It is my mission to get the word out about how incredibly effective M.O.P. is.**"

– *Erin Wetjen, PT, pediatric incontinence specialist,*
Mayo Clinic, Rochester, MN

"**M.O.P. saved my sanity and my daughter's self-esteem.**"

– *Marta Bermudez, Sugar Land, TX*

"**To say this protocol was a life saver is an understatement.**"

– *Verified Amazon purchaser*

Praise for
It's No Accident

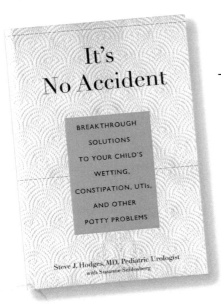

"**Reading this book was a lightbulb moment for me. Dr. Hodges' approach worked for my son!**"

– *Sally Kuzemchak, M.S., R.D., nutritionist and Real Mom Nutrition blogger*

"**This terrific book will help parents better advocate for their kids.**"

– *Shelly Vaziri Flais, M.D., pediatrician, co-editor of*
The Big Book of Symptoms and author of Raising Twins

"***It's No Accident* has completely changed my approach to treating children with urinary issues.**"

– *Daniell Rackley, M.D., Southeastern Urological Center, Tallahassee*

"**Two pediatricians, a GI specialist, and a urologist were not able to help our son. Finally, I found this book and now my son is dry.**"

—*Verified Amazon purchaser*

About the Authors

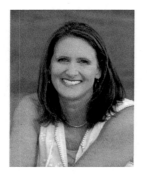

Suzanne Schlosberg

Suzanne is a health and parenting writer who specializes in translating clinical mumbo jumbo into stuff that's fun to read. Years ago, on a mission to achieve a diaper-free household, Suzanne potty-trained her twin boys too early; she used Steve Hodges' methods to undo the damage. The author or co-author of 17 books and countless articles and blog posts, Suzanne manages BedwettingAndAccidents.com, ConstipatedKids.com, and O'Regan Press. Her website is SuzanneSchlosbergWrites.com. Suzanne lives with her husband and boys in Bend, Oregon.

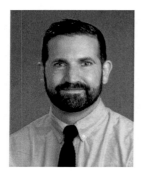

Steve Hodges, M.D.

Steve Hodges is an associate professor of pediatric urology at Wake Forest University School of Medicine and a specialist in childhood toileting issues. He has authored numerous journal articles and co-authored four books with Suzanne Schlosberg. His mission is to shed light on the childhood constipation epidemic and to communicate to families that bedwetting and accidents are never a child's fault. Dr. Hodges lives in Winston-Salem, North Carolina, with his wife and three daughters. He blogs at BedwettingAndAccidents.com and ConstipatedKids.com.

About the Artist

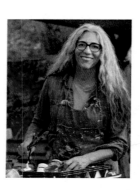

Cristina Acosta

Cristina is a painter and designer known for her lyrical artistry and bold use of color. The author and illustrator of *Paint Happy* and illustrator of *When Woman Became the Sea*, Cristina has taught painting, drawing, and design. Cristina also designs home decor and contributes to interior-design magazines. Though Cristina's daughter is long past potty accidents, Cristina is excited to help children grow up confident and healthy. Cristina divides her time between Palm Springs, California, and Bend, Oregon. Her website is CristinaAcosta.com.

54009793R00024